Yang Sheng:
Nurturing Life

Wisdom and Techniques for Longevity

Jeremy Cornish, LAc.

Contents

Introduction — 2

Section 1: Living Gently — 3
    The Art of Longevity — 4
        The Three Free Therapies — 4
        The Currency of Life — 5
        Running on Fumes — 5
    What to Eat — 6
        The Energetics of Food — 7
        Breakfast Like a King — 7
        Eat When You're Eating — 8
        Postprandial Constitutional — 8
        Congee — 9
        Bone Broth — 10
    Morning Ritual — 11
    Evening Ritual — 11

Section 2: Self Care   12

- Your Constitution (Know Yourself)   13
    - Excess Patterns   13
        - Qi Stagnation   13
        - Blood Stagnation   15
        - Dampness   16
    - Deficiency Patterns   17
        - Qi Deficiency   17
        - Blood Deficiency and Dryness   18
    - Temperature   18
        - Heat   19
        - Cold   19
- How to Stop Getting Sick   20
    - Seasonal Stress   21
    - Lingering Pathogens and Chronic Disease   22

Section 3: Traditional Therapies   23

- Qi Gong   24
    - Triple Burner Breathing   25
- Herbal Formulas   26
    - Adaptogens   26
- Acupuncture   27
    - 7 Ways to Maximize the Effects of Acupuncture   28
    - Side Effects of Acupuncture   29
    - Should You Reschedule Your Next Appointment?   30

Text and Photos Copyright © 2015 Jeremy Cornish, LAc.
All rights reserved.
ISBN-10: 1519232411
ISBN-13: 978-1519232410

Advice in this booklet is not meant to replace a physician.
That being said, please share this information!

Introduction

This booklet is intended to explain the ancient longevity philosophy of Yang Sheng (Nurturing Life), and help you put the principles into practice so that you feel your best.

Please feel free to share this booklet with your friends and family. If you would like extra copies, they are available.

Section 1:
Living Gently

The Art of Longevity

"Yang Sheng" or "nurturing life" is a philosophy of health in Chinese Medicine that recommends learning moderation as opposed to using strict rules to govern how you live. Lifestyle choices regarding what to eat, how to exercise, how much to sleep, when to have sex, how much to work, etc. all add up over time, either to our benefit or detriment. It can be said that the way you feel today is the sum total of every experience and decision you have had so far. The purpose of Yang Sheng is to consciously guide those experiences and decisions to create a long, healthy life.

Yang Sheng practices traditionally involve eating fresh foods that are in season, making time to practice Qi Gong or other internal arts in the morning, enjoying your work, and generally avoiding overtaxing your system. Learning moderation can be summed up by the old Zen adage: "eat when you're hungry; sleep when you're tired."

The Three Free Therapies

In Chinese Medicine, we try to keep in mind what are called the "Three Free Therapies," which include Diet, Exercise, and Rest. The idea is that herbs and acupuncture cost money, but changing lifestyle habits generally doesn't cost much. By addressing dietary irregularities, exercise habits, and encouraging downtime and relaxation, you are priming your system, making acupuncture or any other intervention much more effective.

The Currency of Life

Imagine that when babies are born into the world, they have a savings account of energy (or Qi, pronounced "Chee") to get started on their journey. This savings account comes from the parents, and is referred to as "Jing" or "Jing Qi" in Chinese Medicine. Jing can be translated as "Essence," and it is said to be stored in the Kidneys, as well as the bone marrow. Jing is a deep, finite energy source that each person has had since they were conceived.

Once life begins outside of the womb, there are two other sources of Qi: food and air. Think of the energy that comes from breathing and eating as building up a checking account. This is the energy that we use to function on a day-to-day level. If, for some reason, the energy from food and air isn't enough to get you through a tough day, you begin to draw on your precious reserves of Jing. When the Jing is used up, there is no more Qi in the body, and that's that.

Yang Sheng theory is all about maximizing the energy from food and air, and minimizing stress and energy expenditure so as not to rely on Jing. This is the backbone of Eastern longevity theory.

Running on Fumes

So how do we know when we're using our checking account or dipping into our savings? It's all about developing internal awareness. For example, after a long day, if you sit and close your eyes for a minute, allowing yourself to relax, is it difficult to open them up and get back to your tasks? If so, you're probably tired, which means you should rest, as opposed to dipping into your Jing. You can check in like this any time. If you feel like you are running on fumes, you probably are. This is a sign. When the Qi becomes depleted, other, more obvious signs will show up such as physical symptoms of fatigue, difficulty focusing, low stress threshold, bags under the eyes, pale complexion, etc. Learning not to take on too much at once is a rare skill, but one worth developing.

What to Eat

Whenever a patient asks me what they should be eating, my first answer is always "real food." Real food means that you can identify all the ingredients on the label, or even better, there is no label because the food only has one ingredient (for example, broccoli). Most of the real food is located in the perimeter of the grocery store, not down the aisles. Real food is something that people from one hundred years ago would recognize. Real food often requires that you cook or prepare it. For an excellent read on real food, please see Michael Pollan's book, "Food Rules."

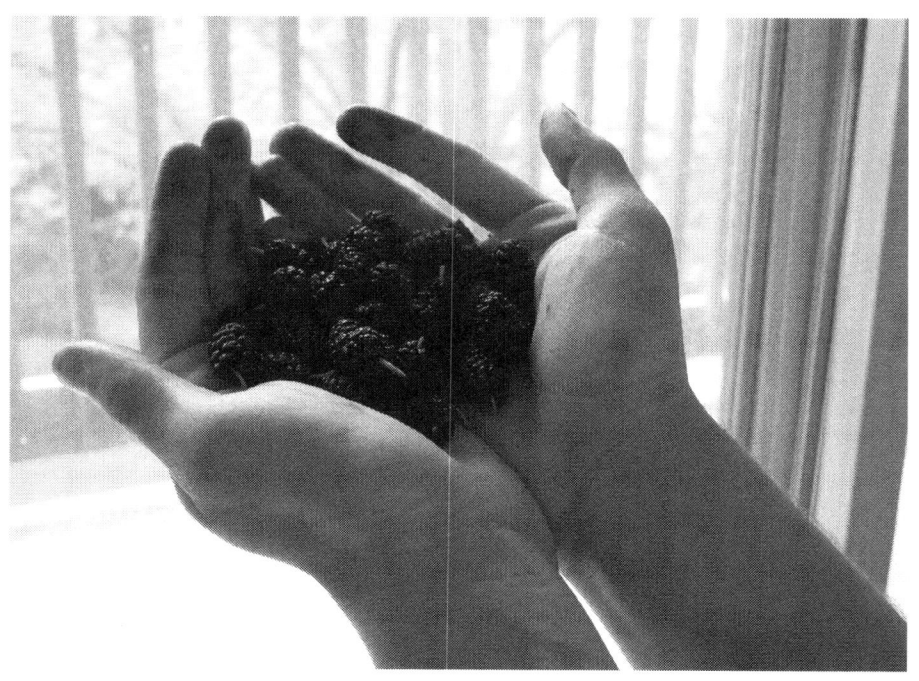

The Energetics of Food

In Chinese Medicine, we recognize the energetic properties of different foods. This is not as grandiose and complex as it may sound. It basically boils down to evaluation based on temperature, moisture, direction, and intensity. For the purposes of this booklet, we can focus on temperature and moisture.

Some foods are cool. Cucumbers, watermelon, and mint are a few examples. Chili peppers, garlic, and onions are hot. Pears and honey are moistening. Dairy products and sweets tend to be damp (too moistening), and can cause phlegm. You might consider the nature of the foods you eat, especially given the time of year (eating watermelons and cucumbers when they're ripe in the summer) to create a balance. If you have a dry throat or a cough, try incorporating more pears and honey.

Eastern nutrition is a sophisticated art, and for the best book I've ever read on the subject, please see "Enlightenweight" by Andrew Miles and Xuelan Qiu.

Breakfast Like a King

There is a saying "eat breakfast like a king, lunch like a prince, and dinner like a pauper." This means the earlier meals should be larger, and dinner should be light. Breakfast is a great chance to load up on healthy foods that will sustain you through most of the workday. Remember, we get a lot of our day-to-day energy from foods. Skipping breakfast is a guaranteed way to run out of energy and be forced to dip into your Jing (energy savings account) to get through the rest of the day.

An excellent guideline for breakfast is to emphasize savory over sweet. You might start with a fresh piece of fruit, then have some eggs, greens, zucchini, tomatoes, and sausage. You could add some roasted potatoes or yams, and a cup of tea. Maybe some sauerkraut. When you emphasize savory, the meal tends to be warmer, with more vegetables and protein. This will give you much more sustained energy than a sweet, cold breakfast of empty carbs.

Cooking your own foods is a lot of work, but it is well worth it. The alarm is going to go off at some point, and no matter when, you're not going to want to get out of bed yet. You might as well set it a half hour earlier. You still won't want to get out of bed, but at least you'll have time to eat a good meal. How you structure your morning sets the tone for the entire day.

Skipping meals teaches your body that food is scarce, which encourages the storage of energy in the form of extra fat.

Eat When You're Eating

One of my teachers used to say this phrase a lot. Our lives are busy, and we have to make time to be present during our meals. In Chinese Medicine, we say that excessive thought injures the digestive system. Eating is not the time for overthinking and multitasking. Your nervous system should be in Parasympathetic mode for optimal digestion, which means your mind must be relaxed. Slow down, chew your food, and enjoy the experience. How you eat is just as important as what you eat. Turn off your phone.

Postprandial Constitutional

Taking a walk after a large meal is an excellent way to facilitate digestion. This should be a nice stroll, not a power walk. The light exercise helps peristalsis (movement of food through the digestive tract), and can prevent gas and bloating. The fresh air helps you relax, and if you have a companion with you, you might find yourself enjoying a conversation instead of the customary "American meditation" (watching TV).

Congee

Congee ("Kon-Jee") is an excellent example of an easily digestible food that is suitable for breakfast, lunch, or dinner. Congee is more of a concept than a specific recipe. The general elements of any congee are overcooked mushy rice, along with additions such as vegetables, herbs, fruits, or even a little meat.
In order for food to be digested and assimilated, our bodies must break it down to a 98.6° soup. Congee is seen as highly nutritious because it is served warm and mushy, thus being easily absorbed without requiring much Qi form the digestive system. How you modify your congee might depend on the season, your constitution, or how you are feeling that particular day. Here is a recipe for a congee that is warming and moistening, perfect for autumn and winter. You may have to go to the Asian grocery for some of the ingredients. Feel free to modify.

Ingredients:
1.5 Cup Jasmine White Rice
1 Can Coconut Milk
3 Cups Water
Small Handful Goji Berries
4-6 Chinese Dates
1 Tbsp Sesame Seeds
Ground Cinnamon
Walnuts

Add the rice, coconut milk, water, gojis, dates, sesame seeds, and a few dashes of cinnamon to a rice cooker or crock pot. Let everything cook until the rice has become a mushy porridge. On a rice cooker, you may have to run it for 2-3 cycles. In a crock pot, the time will depend on the temperature setting.
Scoop the congee into a bowl, top with a few walnuts, and maybe another dash of cinnamon, and enjoy!

Congee is best made in a rice cooker or crock pot, but a pot on the stove works just as well, as long as you can keep an eye on it. Crock pots have the advantage of running in the background so that you can start your congee before bed, and wake up to a hot breakfast with zero effort in the morning.

Bone Broth

Another powerful food to add into your life is bone broth. Homemade beats store bought every time. The benefits of bone broth are being widely explored these days, and it is making something of a comeback in popularity.

To make bone broth, you will need some bones. Some butchers or farmers sell bones just for this purpose. You usually have to ask. Another way to do this is to get a whole chicken, or at least a couple pounds of chicken backs or drumsticks, anything with bones. You could also use beef bones, lamb bones, turkey bones, etc. If you need help sourcing bones, try looking online.

Ingredients:
1lb Bones, 2-3lbs Boney Cuts, or a Whole Chicken
3 Carrots Chopped
3 Stalks Celery Chopped
1 Onion Chopped
1 Tbsp Ground Black Pepper
1 Tbsp Salt
Apple Cider Vinegar
Butter or Olive Oil

You'll also need a skillet, a large pot, a strainer, and a pitcher or small containers Start by sautéing the carrots, onions, and celery in a skillet with butter or oil. Cook until the vegetables are browned. Put the bones/meat/chicken into a large pot, along with the salt and pepper. Add the browned vegetables, and a splash of Apple Cider Vinegar. Add enough water to almost fill the pot, and bring to a boil. Once everything is boiling, reduce the heat, cover, and let it simmer on a low boil for 4-8 hours.

When it's done, wait for it to cool a bit, and then strain out all of the solids and save the broth in glass containers. Broth can be frozen, and will also keep in the fridge for 1-2 weeks.

You can use your broth as a base for other soups (miso, chicken noodle, tom yum, pho, etc), use it instead of water when you make rice (or congee), or simply drink a warm mug every day.

Morning Ritual

The most successful people in the world have one thing in common, they control their mornings. Create a morning ritual for yourself. It doesn't have to be the same each day; simply having some structure in the beginning of the day sets the tone. If you have difficulty finding time to exercise, make time in the morning. If it gets done early, it gets done. An example morning ritual might include drinking a glass of lemon water and eating a little fruit, then spending 10-20 minutes stretching and practicing Qi Gong (see page 24), then preparing a savory breakfast, eating, and starting the day with plenty of fuel and clarity. Or maybe your morning ritual involves putting sweet potatoes in the oven, then taking the dog for a walk while they bake.

Your morning ritual is meant to be a transition between the quiet of sleeping and fasting and the activity of the day. Avoid anything that feels too vigorous too early, and try to make it a gentle transition.

Evening Ritual

Bedtime is another opportunity for ritual to ease the transition from activity to rest. The body is usually more supple in the evening since it has been moving all day. This is a good chance for some gentle yoga, stretching, or Qi Gong. You might practice seated meditation, breathing exercises, self massage, drink some decaffeinated herbal tea, journal, make lists for the next day, or simply read a book. Stay away from bright lights and loud noises (TV, movies, phones, e-books, etc), and of course, no caffeine before bed.

Section 2: Self Care

Your Constitution (Know Yourself)

Each individual has a unique constitution that is the sum total of the internal genetics they came into the world with and the external environment in which they live. In Chinese Medicine we look for big picture patterns and themes as a way to find the root cause of any symptoms that are presenting.

When determining the constitution, one of the first questions to consider is deficiency or excess. In general, do you have too much energy or not enough? Another question to address has to do with temperature. Do you have a tendency towards heat or cold? Also, what are the states of fluid metabolism in the body: is there dryness or dampness? Does the blood contain enough nutrients, and does it circulate well?

Skilled practitioners use a variety of methods including inspecting the pulse, tongue, abdomen, skin, and complexion to determine the overall constitution.

What follows are some basic constitutional pictures. In reality, most people present with a combination of patterns occurring simultaneously, or in different parts of the body.

Excess Patterns

Generally, excess patients tend to be thick, large, and loud. They tend to have a lot of energy, which almost overflows from their body. Extra energy isn't always a good thing. Too much in any area of the body can stagnate. Specific symptoms depend on the individual, and what type of excess they have. Excess can be in the form of Qi Stagnation, Blood Stagnation, or Dampness.

Qi Stagnation

Imagine you are working on your computer when someone you don't really like walks up to interrupt you. They then proceed to criticize your work and shout at you about deadlines. Do you feel what happens in your body? Can you feel your eyes narrow and your shoulders tense? Did your breathing become shallow? Are you clenching your jaw? You've just created a temporary state of Qi Stagnation.

Qi Stagnation most commonly affects the Liver, as that is the organ that is responsible for handling our day-to-day stressors. Liver Qi Stagnation is a widely prevalent pattern in our culture, and typically includes signs and symptoms such as irritability, restlessness, agitation, gas/bloating, tendency towards sighing, neck and shoulder tension, jaw tightness, difficult bowels/IBS, and ulcers, among others. The pulse will have a wiry, tense quality, and high blood pressure is common.

Yang Sheng for Qi Stagnation

We often make choices in search of balance. The tension and internal restlessness that comes with Qi Stagnation often leads people to seek out behaviors that allow them to vent. Some of the most common are smoking cigarettes and drinking alcohol. Both of these habits tend to stir up the Qi, creating a sense of freedom in the short term. Alcohol and cigarettes both add heat to the body, however, which will create more stagnation in the long run. Instead of drinking and smoking, try something safer such as drinking mint tea. Mint is cooling, so it doesn't have the same cumulative side effects as alcohol or cigarettes. Also, it has the effects of mildly moving the Qi, and opening the pores (a light sweat to let off the steam). Mint is also used to calm upset stomachs. A deep breath or a sigh is another way to help disperse Qi Stagnation.

Cigarettes and drinking are also commonly used to treat Qi Stagnation for another reason: community. Find a confidante that doesn't have to be your smoking or drinking buddy. Having a deep conversation with someone close to you (or a professional) can help to sort out your thoughts and relieve your Qi Stagnation.

Qi Stagnation also responds well to exercise. Running, martial arts, weight lifting, yoga, and even taking a leisurely walk can all serve to regulate the Qi of the body. A light sweat is a good sign.

Ultimately, it's best to identify the stressors in life, and do what you can to minimize them or develop more resilience. Even if that means big changes. This is the fine art of listening to your body.

Blood Stagnation

Our blood is responsible for circulating oxygen and nutrients to every cell of the body, as well as bringing warmth, and removing metabolic waste products. Since the blood has so many important jobs to do to keep us alive and well, the quality of blood flow in the body is one of the most important aspects of health. There is a term unique to Chinese Medicine, "Blood Stagnation," which describes a situation where the blood isn't moving as well as it should be, and is often stuck.

Signs of Blood Stagnation include sharp pain, old injuries that linger, cold extremities, poor circulation, cardiac conditions, menstrual problems, depression and emotional trauma, purple marks on the skin, or distended/varicose veins. The tongue also tends to have a purple color, as well as distended purple veins on the underside. The pulse takes on a choppy quality, and the rhythm can be irregular.

Yang Sheng for Blood Stagnation

Blood Stagnation is a common problems in the aging process. Eating well, moving the body gently, and taking time to relax regularly are the best ways to head this off early in life. Ice has a tendency to slow and stagnate the Blood. If you are icing injuries, you may be doing more harm than good over the long term. In most cases, gentle application of heat will help physical injuries heal without stagnation.

If Blood Stagnation is affecting you, the best remedies are actually Chinese Herbal formulas. There are a variety of herbs available depending on the where the stagnation is in the body. Do not try to self-prescribe Chinese Herbs. You definitely want a professional to make the correct formula.

Dampness

In Chinese Medicine, we recognize Dampness as a condition where fluids have built up pathologically in any area of the body. These fluids are stagnant, and need to be excreted through various bodily mechanisms (urination, bowel movements, sweating, etc).

Some symptoms of Dampness include pain (especially joint pain with weather changes), weight gain, swelling, edema, feeling clammy/sweaty, and rashes. Mentally, Dampness can also lead to lethargy, malaise, feeling foggy headed, and a difficulty with change. Dampness can also be present as mucus in the stools, as well as abnormal discharge from any orifice, and can become phlegm in the lungs.

Dampness tends to cause the tongue body to be swollen, often with tooth marks in the sides, and the tongue will often have a thick, slimy, or greasy coating.

Yang Sheng for Dampness

Dampness is primarily seen as a result of an inefficient digestive process. Cold, raw foods are more of a strain on the digestion, and therefore cause more Dampness to build up over time. Additionally, sweet foods tend to have a moistening quality in the body. An excess of sweets in the diet will lead to Dampness. If you are dealing with Dampness, work to minimize dairy products and sugar, as these foods tend to exacerbate the condition. You might eat a little more spicy foods (if your body isn't pathologically hot already) to eliminate some fluids via sweat.

Dampness is a paradox in that there are excess fluids built up in the body, but due to lack of distribution, other body areas are often dehydrated. Food cravings and preferences can often be misleading, as those with Dampness tend to seek out and crave sweets in order to try to bring moisture in, and are often repulsed by liquid foods such as soups, which could actually help the situation. When the body feels soggy already, a bowl of soup is the last thing you want. There is a lot to be said for overcoming the sweet craving, and embracing more appropriate food choices to clear the dampness. If nothing else, make sure you are drinking enough water throughout the day.

Dampness can also be brought on by spending a lot of time in a damp environment. A damp climate, or a subterranean damp living environment can cause the body to take on the dampness in the air. This is a phenomenon that is recognized by Western medicine as well. Those suffering from phlegmy lung diseases such as asthma, and even tuberculosis are often advised to move to a dry climate such as Arizona.

Deficiency Patterns

Generally, deficient patients tend to be thin, small, and soft-spoken. They may feel fatigued, yet have trouble sleeping well. The symptoms depend on the individual, and what type of deficiency (Qi or Blood) they have.

Qi Deficiency

Qi Deficiency is a lack of general energy. This can result in a lack of appetite and poor digestion, as well as feeling tired, exhausted, depressed, or short of breath. Those with Qi Deficiency may have a weak pulse, and the tongue may be puffy, quivering, or have teeth marks in the sides.

Yang Sheng for Qi Deficiency

If this is you, put down the energy drink. To treat Qi Deficiency it's best to create structure in your days so that you eat regularly and maintain balanced blood sugar. Have protein in the mornings at breakfast, and continue to reach for healthy snacks and meals (fruit, nuts, vegetables, etc) throughout the day. One of the main sources of energy is the food we eat. Make sure your choices fuel you. Try to steer your mind away from extraneous thoughts that waste your energy, such as worrying. Also, give yourself permission to take a short nap during the day.

If your Qi is deficient, it is especially important to make sure you are not taking on too many responsibilities. Try not to say "Yes" to every single thing. Get comfortable with down time. You must learn your own limits to prevent further taxation.

Blood Deficiency & Dryness

In Blood Deficiency cases, there is not enough blood to circulate in the body and adequately nourish every cell. This is a pattern that is very common in women. Those with Blood Deficiency will tend to have a pale, thin tongue, pale gums, and thin pulse. Signs of dryness such as dry eyes, dry skin, or brittle hair may be present. Blood Deficiency can cause problems with fertility, sleep, anxiety, and energy level, among others.

Yang Sheng for Blood Deficiency & Dryness

Those with Blood Deficiency do well to stay hydrated, and eat dark, vibrant foods such as kale, chard, black beans, kidney beans, beets, yams, and berries. Red meat such as beef, lamb, and venison (deer) can be very helpful.

Those with Blood Deficiency also need to learn to enjoy down time and not try to fill every moment with an activity or commitment.

Temperature

Another aspect of health that must be taken into consideration is temperature. In Chinese Medicine, we aren't overly concerned with the quantitative temperature (98.6 degrees, etc). What matters most is the subjective experience of heat and cold, and outward observable signs that help to reveal the inner picture. There are herbs and specific acupuncture points that are highly effective at balancing out the internal temperature.

Heat

When there is too much heat in the body, there can be restlessness, insomnia, agitation, redness (eyes, skin, throat, joints, etc), acne, burning sensations, inflammation, strong smells, excessive/abnormal sweating, dark urine, a red tongue, and a rapid pulse. Often the heat in the body will rise and cause headaches. A lot of people with extra heat feel a subjective sensation of warmth, and tend to wear light clothing.

Yang Sheng for Heat

If you have too much heat in the body, consider cooling foods such as cucumbers, watermelon, salads, and mint tea. Avoid excessively spicy foods and smoking or alcohol. Exercise regularly to facilitate sweating.

Cold

When there is too much cold in the body (not enough heat), there can be lethargy, low libido, infertility, pale or bluish coloring, weight gain, frequent clear urination, low appetite, indigestion, constipation or loose watery stools, clamminess or a lack of sweat, a pale tongue and a slow pulse. Most cold people will feel cold internally, and often dress in heavier clothing or more layers.

Yang Sheng for Cold

If you have too much cold in the body, consider warming foods such as garlic, ginger, onions, and chili peppers. Avoid cold or raw foods such as ice cream, salads, and smoothies (no matter how "healthy" they're supposed to be). Exercise regularly to keep the body warm. Try to use a sauna or hot tub regularly.

How to Stop Getting Sick

In Chinese Medicine we recognize the body as a kingdom, which is constantly under attack by the forces of the environment (heat, cold, dryness, dampness, wind). The Wei Qi ("way chee") is the energy that is said to guard the exterior of the body, protecting the boundaries from invasion. When the Wei Qi is strong, we have a healthy immune system, and the invaders (heat, cold, dryness, dampness, and wind, as well as viruses, bacteria, etc) don't have a chance to penetrate to the interior of the body. When the Wei Qi is weak (from overwork, stress, poor nutrition, lack of exercise, genetics, etc) the boundaries are vulnerable, and we get sick. A careful look at the symptoms will tell which of the forces (heat, cold, dryness, dampness, wind) are causing the illness and how best to resolve it.

Catching a Cold
The concept of external climactic forces is not entirely foreign to our culture. We have a term "Catching a Cold." In Chinese Medicine, we can see that excessive cold has penetrated the body when there are symptoms such as chills, slight fever (the body trying to warm itself for balance), sweating (the body trying to push the cold back out), achy joints (the cold settling into the joints and obstructing the flow), sinus pressure, clear nasal discharge, and fatigue (cold slowing the body down).

Yang Sheng for External Cold
One way to protect against cold entering the body is to help your Wei Qi by wearing appropriate clothing to guard against invasion. A scarf over the nape of the neck is highly recommended when it's cold out. Also, don't expose yourself to cold while the pores are open (sweating). If possible, don't sit directly under air conditioning vents for a prolonged time.

If you are already experiencing Cold invasion, your best move is to sweat it out. Spend time in a sauna, hot tub, or steam room. Eat pungent foods such as ginger tea, garlic, chili peppers, or miso soup with green onions.
Of course Chinese Herbs will be a big help, as well as therapies that open the pores such as cupping or gua sha.

Catching Heat

In Chinese Medicine, not everyone who "has a cold" actually has cold. Often there is heat that needs to be treated. Externally contracted heat includes symptoms such as sore, red throat, high fever, sweating, mania (heat affecting the mind), insomnia, thick yellow or green phlegm (heat "cooks down" the phlegm and darkens it), dark urine, and thirst.

Yang Sheng for External Heat

Heat pathogens are said to enter the body through the mouth. That's because heat usually begins by causing a sore throat. For sore throat, mint tea, coconut water, or a salt water gargle (do not swallow) can be helpful. If there is high fever, and the heat is rising to the head, a cool wet towel on the forehead or nape of the neck can bring some relief. Another way to regulate the temperature dynamic is to warm the feet. This could be done via a warm foot bath, or wrapping a heating pad around the feet. Some people even put cayenne pepper or cinnamon on the bottoms of the feet. This helps to bring the heat down and create the ideal thermal scenario of "cool head, warm feet."

Seasonal Stress

Transitions create stress on the body, which weakens the immune system. It is for this reason that we often get sick during seasonal changes. A great way to use acupuncture and herbs as part of your Yang Sheng is to schedule a session quarterly, at the change of the season. There are specific techniques that can help the body transition to the next season with strength.

If you are someone who knows that you get sick often, or at the change of seasons, there are herbs you can take proactively to help build your Wei Qi. If a pathogen does manage to penetrate your defenses, it is important to make sure it is fully resolved so that it doesn't linger.

Seasonal treatments are also a highly beneficial practice for kids, especially when you consider the times of year that they tend to get sick (back to school, holidays, springtime, etc). Yang Sheng is all about prevention.

Lingering Pathogens and Chronic Diseases

A lot of people get sick in predictable patterns. Here is a common one:

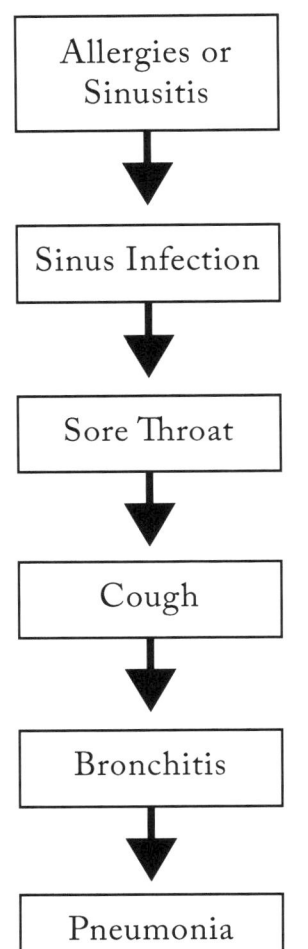

In this example it is easy to see that as the pathogen moves more deeply into the body, the symptoms become more and more severe. In Chinese Medicine, we use different herbal combinations depending on the type of pathogen (Heat, Cold, etc) and how deeply it has penetrated the body. It is extremely important to lead the pathogen back out to prevent "Lingering Pathogens."

A Lingering Pathogen is a situation where an unwelcome foreign force has penetrated the normal defenses of the body, and now hides out (lingers) inside. Whenever the immune system (Wei Qi) is low, the pathogen takes advantage and flares up.

A lot of complex medical conditions such as fibromyalgia and chronic fatigue syndrome may present with a Lingering Pathogen component. The western understanding of viruses that lie dormant in nerves and flare up during times of stress (shingles, herpes, MS, Lyme's) also clearly fit into the Lingering Pathogen model.

Treating Lingering Pathogens

If you think you may have a Lingering Pathogen, it is best to seek treatment from a professional Acupuncturist.

Section 3: Traditional Therapies

Qi Gong

"Qi Gong" ("Chee Gong") is a Chinese term that loosely translates as "energy cultivation" or "energy practice." It is a very broad term covering all sorts of exercises and meditations that promote relaxation, flexibility, internal strength, longevity, and peace of mind.

The benefits of a regular Qi Gong practice are profound. As with any exercise regimen, you ought to experience better sleep, weight loss, and increased energy. Qi Gong also has a tendency to provide pain relief, and emotional regulation. Working with Qi tends to bring a sense of calm and peace, and guiding the energy through the body helps to promote healing. In Chinese Medicine, we say pain is due to lack of free flow. Improving the Qi flow (and blood circulation) in the painful area can sometimes make all the difference.

Another common benefit of regular Qi Gong practice is the increase of synchronistic events in your life. I have noticed this myself, and many of the students I've worked with have made similar observations. Coincidences seem to come up very frequently, and "manifesting" practices tend to become quicker and easier. This may be due to an enhanced personal vibration rippling into the universe, or simply the fact that a more calm, clear mind can more easily recognize the coincidences that are always happening around us. Either way, life just seems to flow better with regular Qi Gong practice.

You may also notice your personality changes a bit. Qi Gong practice promotes a feeling of neutrality and acceptance. Generally, those who meditate regularly have less turbulent emotional ups and downs, and are more able to stay centered through the twists and turns of life. Due to the meditative nature of Qi Gong, most practitioners tend to be bothered less and less by personal dramas. External events tend to have less emotional impact as the internal center becomes stronger.

Triple Burner Breathing

Begin by standing comfortably with the spine long and the knees slightly bent.

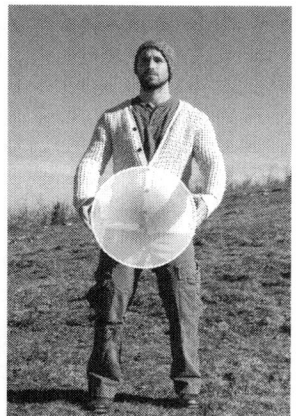

When you're ready, bring the hands in front of the lower abdomen and let the centers of the palms face each other. Imagine there is a ball of energy between the hands. As you inhale, allow the hands to move away from each other a couple inches, and feel the ball expand to fill the new space. On the exhalation, reverse the motion, compressing the ball back to its original size, charging it with energy. With some practice, you'll begin to sense a density in the space between the hands. Repeat at least nine times.

The Energy Ball

Once you have built some energy between the hands, you can practice Triple Burner Breathing:

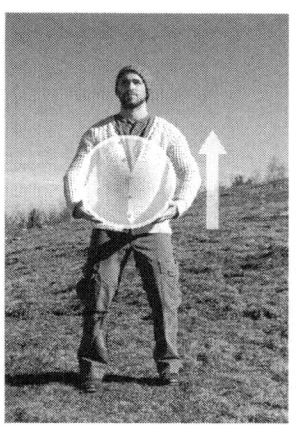 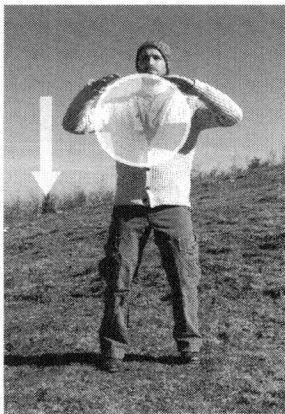

1. As you inhale, turn the palms toward the sky, lifting the ball up to the top of the chest.

2. As you exhale, turn the palms toward the ground, lowering the ball back to the abdomen.

Repeat at least 9 times, then stand for a moment with the arms at the sides, letting your mind rest while you direct your attention inwards and notice the sensations in your body.

For much more comprehensive and detailed Qi Gong instruction, please see my book, "Mountain Shadow Qi Gong," or attend a class or workshop.

Herbal Formulas

Chinese Herbs help regulate the body by adjusting parameters such as heat/cold, dryness/moisture, excess/deficiency within the body. They are much more powerful and focused than foods, and it is extremely important to have an experienced professional create a formula for you.

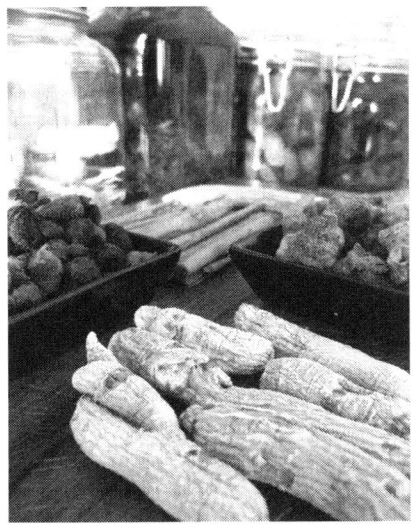

Herbs can be taken internally (as teas, pills, tinctures, or powders) or applied topically to the skin (as poultices, powders, oils, balms, or liniments).

External application is often used for injuries (chronic or acute), as well as skin conditions such as rashes, acne, burns, tinea/fungus, poison ivy, and eczema.

Adaptogens

There is a special category of herbs that have systematic benefits and promote good health. These herbs are called "Adaptogens" as they help the body adapt to the stresses of life. Ginseng is one of the most famous Adaptogens. Others include Goji Berries, Wu Wei Zi, Dang Shen, Jiao Gu Lan, and many more.

Some Adaptogens have certain specialties, such as benefiting mood, treating altitude sickness, increasing energy, or boosting sexual function. If you choose to incorporate Adaptogens into your life, you can generally experiment for yourself, or seek a professional opinion to determine the best place to start, depending on your goals.

For information on Adaptogens, I recommend Ron Teegarden's book "Chinese Tonic Herbs."

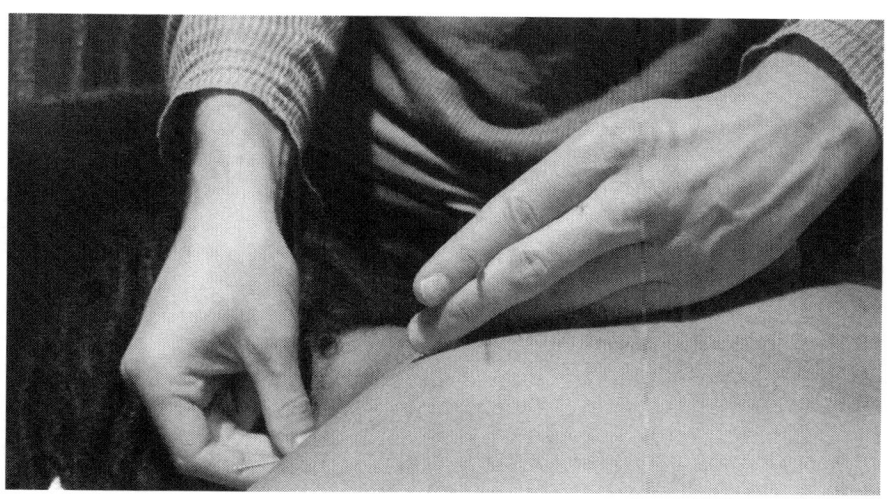

Acupuncture

Acupuncture works by utilizing the Qi, or vital energy that is inherent in your body. There is no medicine on the needles. The needles only work to stimulate natural processes that your body already has in place.

Acupuncture can be safely and effectively used for almost any health condition, especially:

- Allergies
- Anxiety
- Cancer Support
- Chronic Diseases
- Depression
- Fasciitis
- Fatigue
- Hormonal
- Immune
- Indigestion
- Insomnia
- Migraines
- Pain/Injuries
- Pediatrics
- Pregnancy
- Stress

7 Ways to Maximize the Effects of Acupuncture

1. **Eat Something Beforehand.** Acupuncture works by directing the energy in your body in specific ways. If you have a little food in your belly, then there's more energy to use for your treatment. We get hungry when we are in need of more fuel. Acupuncture works so much better when you bring more Qi to the table.

2. **Avoid Caffeine Beforehand.** The only thing worse than acupuncture on an empty stomach is acupuncture on a stomach full of nothing but coffee. Acupuncture works to help you relax by increasing a neurotransmitter in your brain called Adenosine. This is a neurotransmitter that makes you feel calm and restful. Biochemically, Caffeine doesn't give you energy, it just blocks Adenosine, so you don't feel tired. Mixing Acupuncture with a lot of Caffeine is like breaking even in terms of Adenosine.

3. **Less Strenuous Activity.** Please don't think of your body as fragile immediately after an acupuncture session, though it is advisable to exercise on the lighter side for the rest of the day. We are directing your energy to specific places. Try not to spend all of it lifting pieces of iron. Acupuncture tends to have an excellent pain relieving effect. Your injured body part might feel stronger than it actually is immediately after acupuncture. Please don't push it.

4. **Incorporate the 3 Free Therapies.** See page 3 of this booklet. Also, don't forget the bonus fourth free therapy: Fun. Do something that makes you laugh. That is very good for the Qi.

5. **Arrive on Time.** This almost goes without saying, but it's better to have the whole appointment to let the needles do their work.

6. **Strategic Scheduling.** It's best to think of acupuncture as a process rather than as isolated treatments. Your acupuncturist should be able to help you figure out a schedule to keep the treatments regular. Often this schedule starts with a higher frequency in the beginning, then a taper to wean you off as your condition improves. The treatment plan is based on your acupuncturist's experience with cases like yours and what has worked the best in the past.

7. **Turn off your Phone.** Yep. You're lying on the table, your mind is finally calming down, and you begin to slip into a blissful, half-waking dreamlike state. The Adenosine release is kicking in. Then BUZZZ your phone jabs you awake. Better to turn it off. Turn everything off. When you are on the table it is a chance to not have to be in charge of everything in your life. How rare are these moments?

Side Effects of Acupuncture

As a medical treatment, acupuncture is remarkably safe and free of side effects. That being said, it's not uncommon for minor side effects in the areas where the needles were, such as itchiness, redness, slight swelling, bruising, soreness, and other sensations.

These effects are all typically harmless and self-limiting. Some (such as itchiness, redness, and soreness) can also be seen as a positive sign of progress in certain cases.

Common Side Effects of Acupuncture
• Better Sleep
• More Energy
• Mental Calmness
• Giddiness
• Relaxation
• Pain Relief
• Feeling Hungry
• Balanced Mood

The most common side effects people notice after acupuncture tend to be positive, and speak to the holistic nature of the treatment.

After acupuncture, patients commonly report better sleep, more energy, mental calmness, giddiness, relaxation, general decrease of aches and pains, feeling hungry (increased metabolism), and balanced mood.

In short, regulating the Qi makes you feel good.

Should you reschedule your next acupuncture appointment?

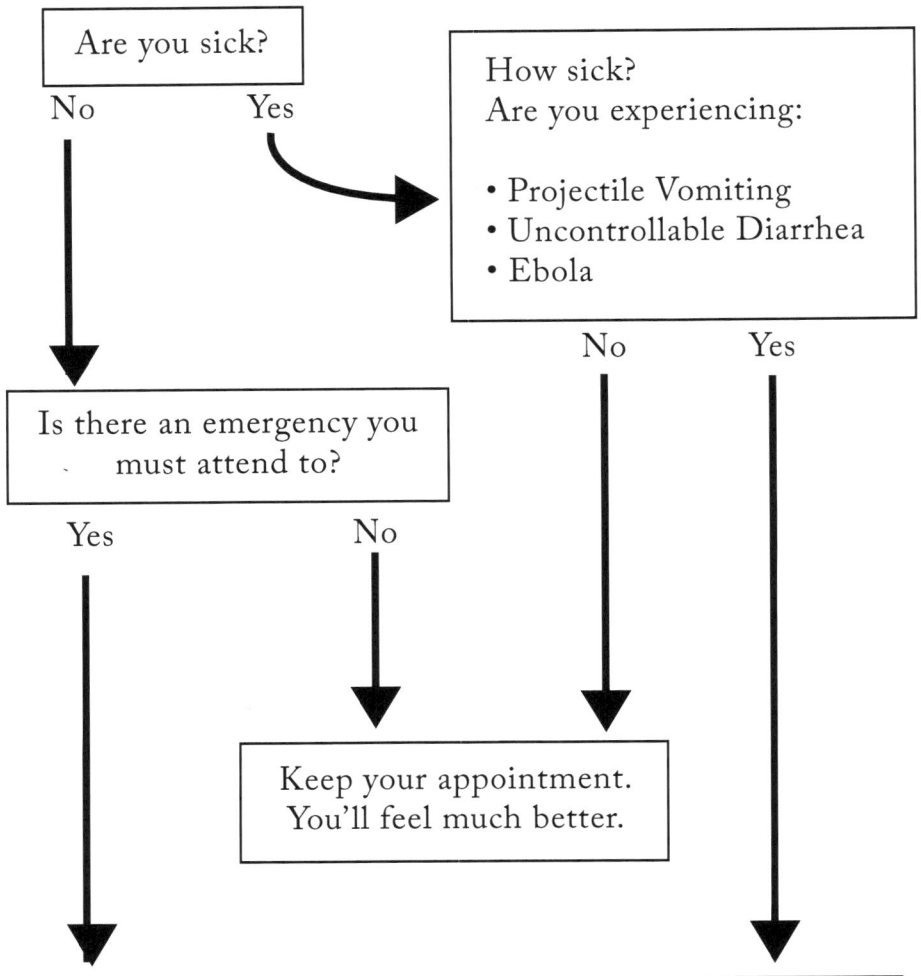

Made in the USA
Las Vegas, NV
17 October 2020